Laila is a school student, who is passionate about all things sports and health related. And so, she started pursuing first aid and safety in order to expand her knowledge and be a more active member in her community. She is very family and community oriented and therefore, has a passion for sharing her knowledge with others. She hopes that this book will be of help for people to grasp the basics of first aid.

This book is dedicated to my grandparents, Prof. Dr El-Sayed Mohamed Abdelbary and Prof. Dr Fadia Mohamed Amin Ghali. You are my inspiration.

Laila Abdelbary

STAY ALERT: CHILDREN'S GUIDE TO BASIC FIRST AID

AUSTIN MACAULEY PUBLISHERS™
LONDON * CAMBRIDGE * NEW YORK * SHARJAH

Copyright © Laila Abdelbary 2022

The right of Laila Abdelbary to be identified as author of this work has been asserted by Laila Abdelbary in accordance with Federal Law No. (7) of UAE, Year 2002, Concerning Copyrights and Neighboring Rights.

All rights reserved. No part of this publication may be reproduced, stored in a retrieval system, or transmitted in any form or by any means, electronic, mechanical, photocopying, recording, or otherwise, without the prior permission of the publishers.

Any person who commits any unauthorized act in relation to this publication may be liable to legal prosecution and civil claims for damages.

The age group that matches the content of the books has been classified according to the age classification system issued by the Ministry of Culture and Youth.

This book is intended for informational purposes only. To perform first aid, a person needs to be trained and qualified by an appropriate medical entity specialised in this field.

ISBN – 9789948044710 – (Paperback)
ISBN – 9789948044727 – (E-Book)

Application Number: MC-10-01-1734021
Age Classification: E

First Published 2022
AUSTIN MACAULEY PUBLISHERS FZE
Sharjah Publishing City
P.O Box [519201]
Sharjah, UAE
www.austinmacauley.ae
+971 655 95 202

Table of Contents

First Aid	9
How To Get Help and Describe The Situation	10
Getting Help	11
CPR	12
Choking	14
Burns	16
Bleeding and Shock	17
Muscle, Bone and Joint Injuries	19
Allergies	20
Asthma Attacks	22
Recovery Position	23
Golden Rules of First Aid	24
Activities Word search	25
Activities Match the Word to Its Definition	26
Activities Color In These First Aid Tools	27
Activities Color In These First Aid Tools	28
Sources	29

First Aid

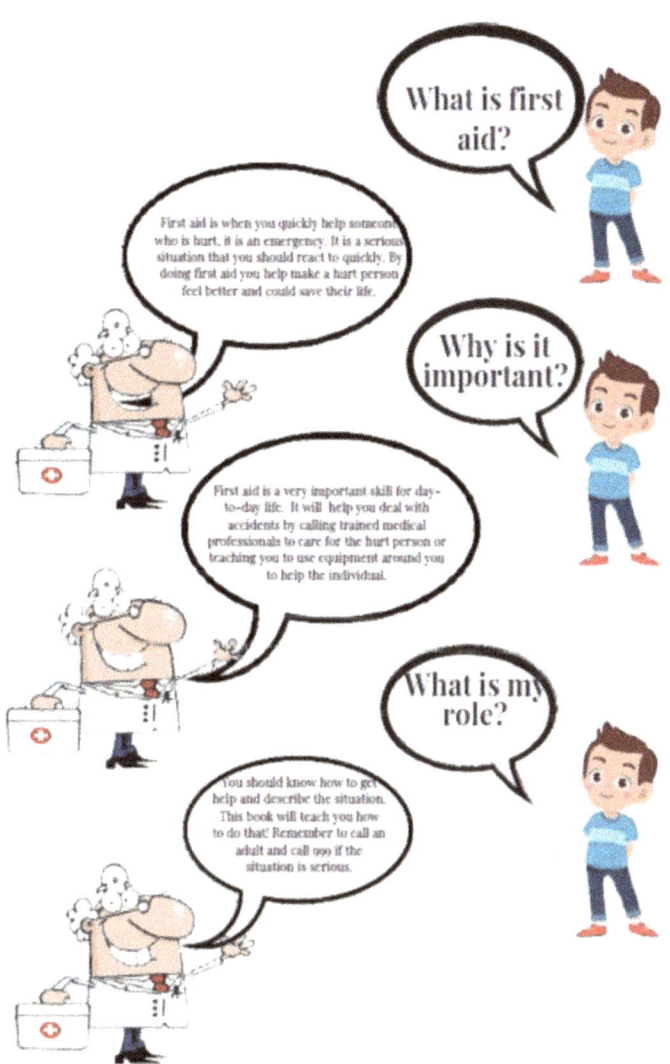

How To Get Help and Describe The Situation

Usually, the most important thing you can do in a crisis is call for help. To do this **open a phone keypad and call 999.** But it is important to never use emergency numbers for play or out of curiosity.

When to call?

In order to check how serious, the incident is following the **DRAB** procedure.

Basic assessment comes hand in hand with calling for help.

Danger:- Take a moment to make sure it is safe to approach the injured person: are there any hazards such as electrical wires, damaged structures, moving vehicles, or falling objects? If the surroundings are dangerous, get help right away before trying to help.

Response:- Talk to the injured person. Do they answer questions? Do they appear to be awake or unconscious? The emergency operator (person on the phone) will ask you how they respond.

Airway:- If unconscious, gently tip their head back to make sure the tongue is not blocking their airway.

Breathing

If there is no adult around to help you make the assessment, it is always best to call 999.

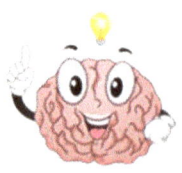

Getting Help

Call 999 In an Emergency
Ask For

Police   Ambulance   Fire

Give them:
- Your name
- Your address
- Phone number
- And what happened

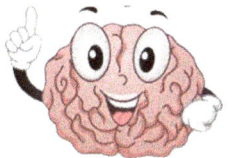

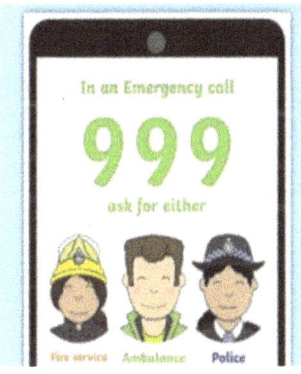

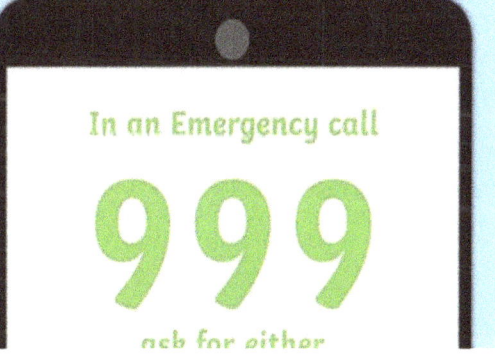

CPR

CPR helps to stimulate the heart and causes it to start beating again.
If someone is **unconscious** and you need to check if they are breathing…
Look, **listen**, and **feel** for breaths

Look   Listen   Feel

Make sure to tell an adult and call 999

If they are not breathing, Start CPR until help arrives

Chest compressions: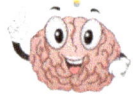

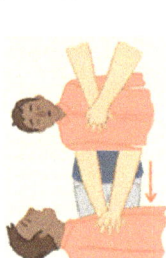

- Interlock your hands at the center of their chest.
- Push hard and fast, about twice per second.
- Repeat cycles of 30 compressions.

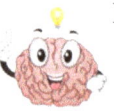 REMEMBER: Look, listen, and feel for breaths

Glossary

Unconscious = when a person is unable to respond to people and activities

Choking

It is when the **airway** is partly or completely blocked, this cuts off oxygen to the brain. Some **symptoms** you may see is that they struggle to breath properly. They may be able to clear it by coughing but if not tell an adult and call 999 immediately.

You are having dinner with your mum when she starts choking, what do you do?

Step One: **Cough it out•** Encourage her to keep coughing

Step Two: **Slap it out•** Give 5 sharp back blows between the shoulder blades. **Turn your palms forward and hit the heel of your palm against her back•** Check her mouth each time.

Step Three: **Squeeze it out•** Give 5 abdominal thrusts.

- Check her mouth each time. **Place your arms around her waist and bend her forward. And then pull your arms sharply inward** only do this step if you're able to reach around the person.

Step four: Call 999 for emergency help

- Repeat steps 2 and 3 until help arrives.

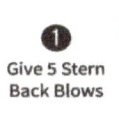 Give 5 Stern Back Blows 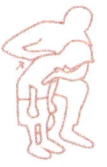 Give 5 Abdominal Thrusts

 Continue by Alternating Back Blows and Abdominal Thrusts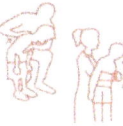

Glossary

Symptom = A sign which could indicate a more serious condition.

Airway = the passage by which air reaches a person's lungs.

REMEMBER:

Hit their back

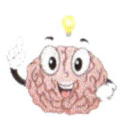

Burns

A burn is a type of injury to skin. It is caused by heat, cold, electricity, chemicals, **friction**, or radiation (like sunburn).

Minor Burns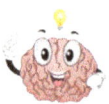

1. Hold burn under cool running water for **at least 10-20 minutes.**
2. Remove clothing or jewelry around the burn, **unless stuck to the burn**.
3. Cover lengthways with cling film.
4. stay around the injured individual and get medical advice.

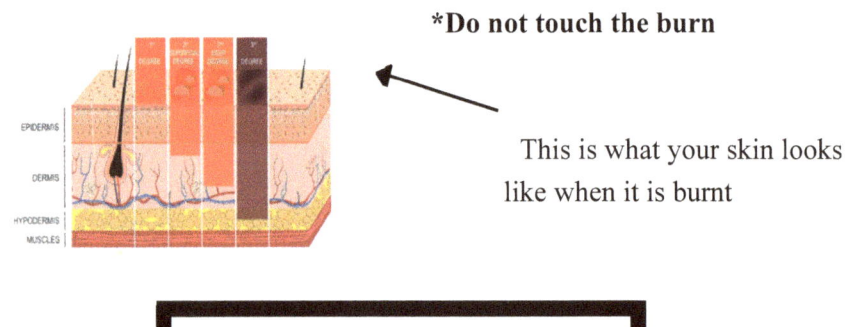

*Do not touch the burn

This is what your skin looks like when it is burnt

Glossary

Friction =It is like a dragging motion. Resisting the motion of a fluid across the surface of a body which results in a burn.

16

Bleeding and Shock

If someone has a bad bleed...

Press firmly on the bleed using some clean fabric such as a piece of cotton, towel, or item of clothing **and keep pressing**. To help slow down the bleeding raise the injured area so that it's higher than their chest.

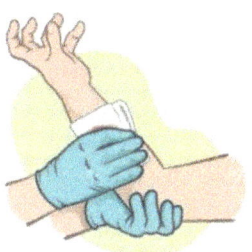

So now when your friend falls down at the playground and starts bleeding, what will you do?

Shock

This happens if the body begins to lose large amounts of blood. If this occurs immediately call 999.

Treat the person for shock by making them lie down with their head low, their legs raised and wrap them with a blanket.

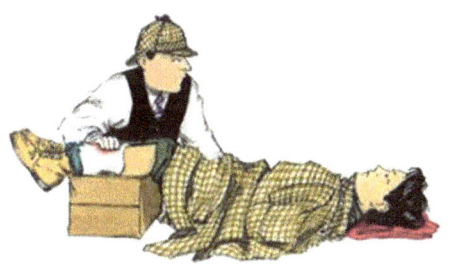

Nosebleeds

- Help the person lean their head forward.
- get them to pinch the soft part of their nose for 10 minutes.

- Remember press hard on bleeds.
- Lean forward if you have a nose bleed.
- Call 999 if the individual looks tired and lay them down with their legs raised wrapped with a blanket.

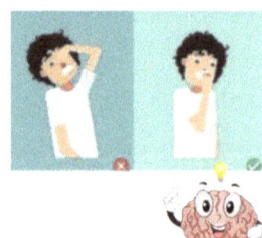

Glossary

Injury=Damage to the body/ something that it hurt due to a form of accident.

Muscle, Bone and Joint Injuries

Sprains and strains

Signs and symptoms = Bruising, swelling, and pain.

Use the RICE method

R – Rest –> Avoid use of injured area.

I – Ice –> Apply ice or cold pack to reduce swelling.

C – Compression –> Wrap the injured joint with an elastic bandage to avoid further injury and reduce swelling.

E – Elevate – >Reduce swelling.

Fractures (broken bones)

Signs and symptoms =

More painful than sprains or strains, the injured area may look different.

- **Immobilize** the area – make the person comfortable so they can **keep the injured part still.**
- Don't try to move them unless they are in danger.
- Call 999 for help if there is no adult.

REMEMBER:

Keep it still and support it until help arrives.

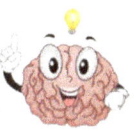

Glossary

Immobilize = prevent someone or something from moving as normal.

Allergies

An allergic reaction may occur if someone comes in contact with an allergen. Allergen's may be harmless to most people. Some environments, food, or even medications may be allergens. Talk to your friends and find out what they are allergic to!

If someone has an allergic reaction they may have trouble breathing. In this case call 999 immediately and say ANAPHYLAXIS (ana-fil-ax-is). If they stop breathing follow the steps of CPR.

Signs and symptoms =

AIRWAY
Persistent cough, hoarse voice, difficulty swallowing, swollen tongue

BREATHING
Difficult or noisy breathing, wheeze or persistent cough

CONSCIOUSNESS
Persistent dizziness, p or floppy, suddenly sle collapse, unconscious

Until help arrives lay them flat with their legs raised.

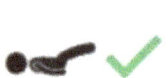  

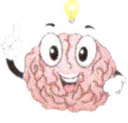

if someone experiences an allergic reaction, call 999 immediately and on the phone say anaphylaxis. Talk and make sure you or anyone who has severe allergies carries around an EpiPen.

Glossary

Adrenaline auto generator=sometimes referred to as an allergic reaction a dose of adrenaline which treats anaphylaxis

Asthma Attacks

Asthma occurs when your airways narrow and swell and may produce extra mucus. As a result it makes breathing difficult and triggers coughing, a whistling sound (wheezing) when you breathe out, and shortness of breath.

Signs and symptoms =
wheezing, coughing, shortness of breath, and panic.

How to help

- Get the person to rest comfortable, sitting down.
- Help the person to use their reliever inhaler straight away
- If they're no better after a few minutes, get them to take one or two puffs of their inhaler every minute until they've had 10 puffs.
- If they are still struggling, call 999

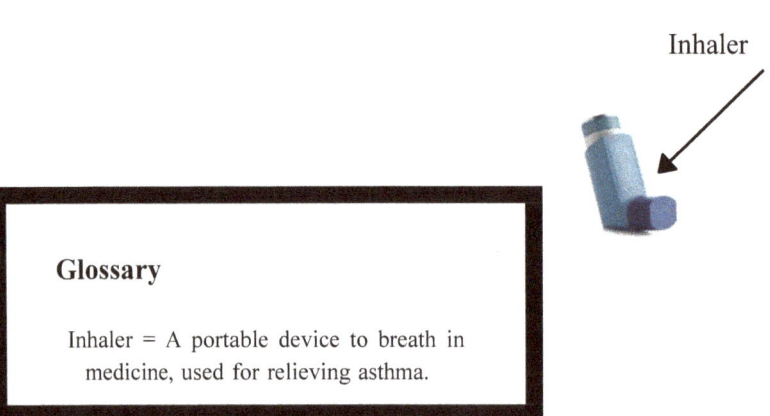

Inhaler

Glossary

Inhaler = A portable device to breath in medicine, used for relieving asthma.

Recovery Position

The recovery position prevents an individual from choking when they are unconscious until help arrives.

Only put someone in this position if you can hear, see, or feel that they are breathing. Make sure they are not injured. Moving someone who is injured may hurt them more.

1. If the person is laying on their back, kneel on the floor at their side.
2. Extend the arm nearest to you at a right angle to their body with their palm facing up.
3. Take their other arm and fold it so the back of their hand rests on the cheek closest to you, and hold it in place.

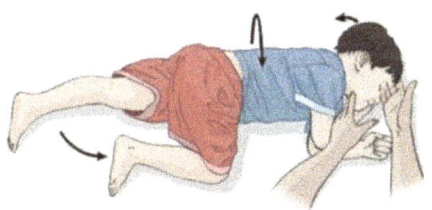

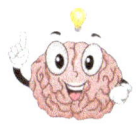

REMEMBER:
Roll on side and tilt head back

Golden Rules of First Aid

Stay calm
1. Call 999 in an emergency.
2. On the phone tell the medical expert as much as you possibly can about the accident.
3. If surrounding is unsafe don't approach the individual.
4. Reassure the hurt person.
5. Ensure hands are clean before dealing with wounds and burns to avoid infection.

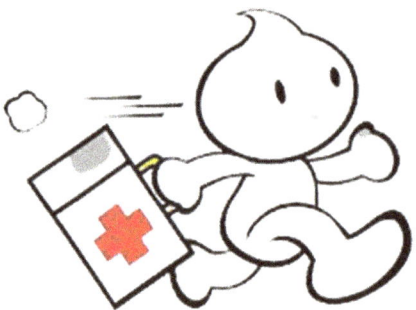

Activities
Word search

Name: _____

First aid

```
P  S  H  O  C  K  T  D  E  H  Y  D  R  A  T  E  D  C
M  M  L  A  L  L  E  R  G  I  E  S  R  F  O  Q  J  R
U  D  E  P  I  P  E  N  C  N  H  E  A  T  N  E  M  E
S  S  L  K  C  H  O  C  K  I  N  G  Y  K  M  F  X  C
C  F  I  V  E  A  N  D  F  I  V  E  H  L  L  W  A  O
L  C  H  E  S  T  C  O  M  P  R  E  S  S  I  O  N  V
E  G  X  D  E  F  I  B  R  I  L  L  A  T  I  O  N  E
C  J  H  Y  P  O  T  H  E  R  M  I  A  P  M  H  B  R
S  P  S  V  B  R  O  K  E  N  X  J  F  T  K  E  O  Y
N  J  R  Z  U  N  C  O  N  S  C  I  O  U  S  L  N  O
B  J  O  I  N  T  F  C  X  B  H  B  U  R  N  P  E  K
M  Y  W  H  E  I  N  J  U  R  Y  S  R  G  S  L  C  R
```

Find the following words in the puzzle.
Words are hidden → ↓ and ↘ .

ALLERGIES
BONE
BROKEN
BURN
CHEST COMPRESSION
CHOCKING
CPR
DEFIBRILLATION
DEHYDRATED
EPIPEN
FIVE-AND-FIVE
HEAT
HELP
HYPOTHERMIA
INJURY
JOINT
MUSCLE
RECOVERY
SHOCK
UNCONSCIOUS

Activities
Match the Word to
Its Definition

Allergic reaction	caused by someone reacting badly due to sensitivities to substances called allergens. It occurs when it comes into contact with skin, nose, eyes, respiratory tract. They can be inhaled into the lungs, swallowed, or injected.
Asthma attack	A state when a person is unable to respond to people and activities.
Unconscious	A serious situation requiring immediate attention.
Shock	the airways become swollen and inflamed. Breathing becomes more difficult due to added mucus. During an attack, you may cough, wheeze and have trouble breathing.
CPR	Damage to the skin caused by heat.
Fracture	A physical or mental feature which is regarded as indicating a condition.
Burn	A broken bone
Emergency	helps to stimulate the heart and causes it to start beating again. It is a lifesaving technique useful in many emergencies, where someone's breathing or heartbeat has stopped.
Symptoms	Caused by organs not getting enough blood or oxygen. It can be a result of heatstroke, blood loss, an allergic reaction, severe infection, poisoning, or severe burns

Activities
Color In These First Aid Tools

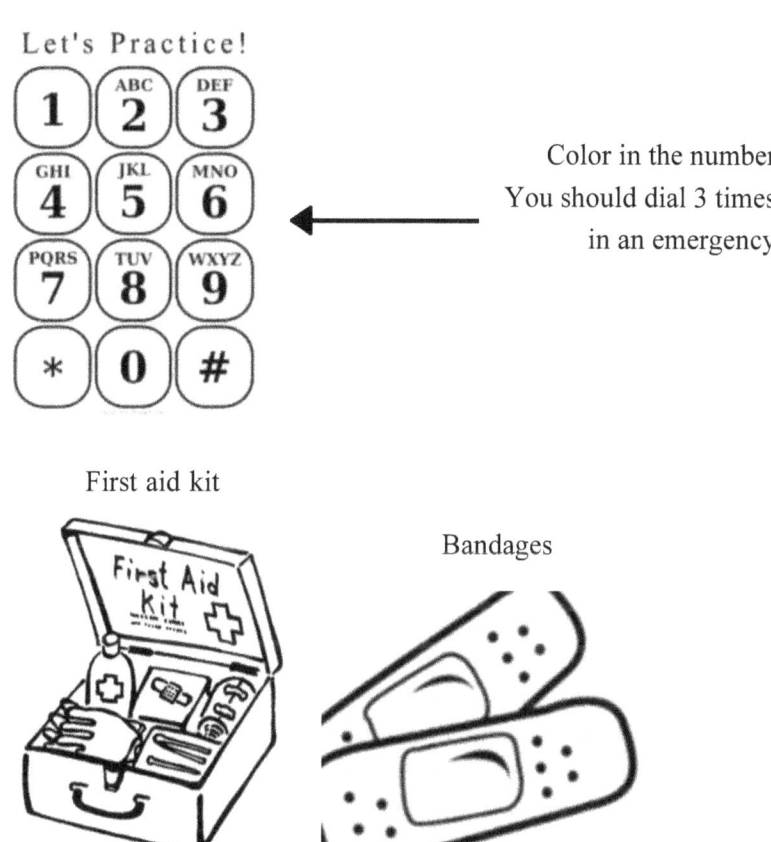

Color in the number
You should dial 3 times
in an emergency

First aid kit

Bandages

Activities
Color In These
First Aid Tools

Thermometer

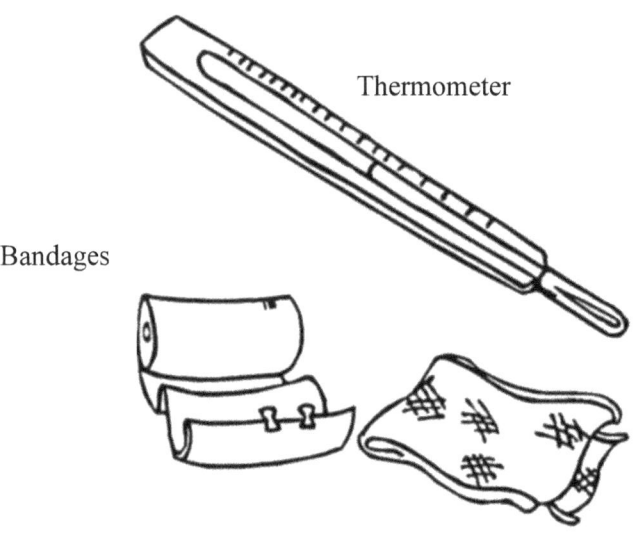

Bandages

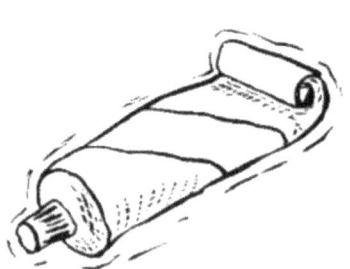

Ointment

Ambulance

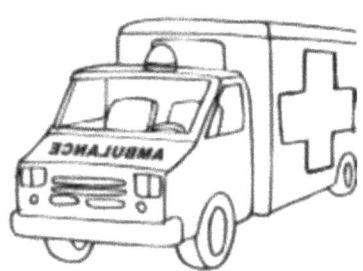

Sources

1. All the First Aid Stuff That's Changed Since You First Learned It. Lifehacker, 12 Nov. 2015, lifehacker.com/all-the-first-aid-stuff-thats-changed-since-you-first-l-1742121480.
2. Blok, Barbara, et al. Mc Graw Hill Education, 2016, First aid for the emergency medicine boards, First Aid for the Emergency Medicine Board (PDF Drive).pdf.
3. Bobek, Eliza, and Barbara Tversky. "Creating Visual Explanations Improves Learning." Cognitive Research: Principles and Implications, Springer International Publishing, 2016, www.ncbi.nlm.nih.gov/pmc/articles/PMC5256450/.
4. Clark, Daniel. "What Are the 5 Main Aims of First Aid?: First Aid." Engage in Learning, 11 Feb. 2020, www.engageinlearning.com/faq/health-safety/first-aid/what-are-the-5-main-aims-of-first-aid/.
5. First Aid Online Classes: Online First Aid. Red Cross, www.redcross.org/take-a-class/first-aid/first-aid-training/first-aid-online.
6. First Aid Skills Everybody Should Know, www.cprcertified.com/blog/first-aid-skills-everybody-should-know.
7. Furst, John. "The Aims of First Aid – the Three Ps." First Aid for Free, 23 Aug. 2017, www.firstaidforfree.com/the-aims-of-first-aid-three-ps/.
8. Gutierrez, K. (n.d.). Studies Confirm the Power of Visuals in eLearning. Retrieved October 6, 2020, from https://www.shiftelearning.com/blog/bid/350326/studies-confirm-the-power-of-visuals-in-elearning.
9. Gutierrez, Karla. 6 Ways Color Psychology Can Be Used to Design Effective eLearning, www.shiftelearning.com/blog/bid/348188/6-Ways-Color-Psychology-Can-Be-Used-to-Design-Effective-eLearning.

10. Hammett, Emma, and Name *. "First Aid Saves Lives – Ten Powerful Reasons to Learn First Aid This Year." First Aid for Life, 17 Feb. 2020, firstaidforlife.org.uk/first-aid/.
11. History of CPR.Cpr.heart.org, cpr.heart.org/en/resources/history-of-cpr.
12. Lombardi, Lisa. "13 Common First Aid Mistakes Everyone Makes." The Healthy, The Healthy, 18 May 2020, www.thehealthy.com/first-aid/common-first-aid-mistakes/.
13. Mohan, Janet, editor. FIRST AID MANUAL. 5th ed., Sarah Larter, 2014.
14. Order of Importance. Reading Worksheets, www.ereadingworksheets.com/text-structure/patterns-of-organization/order-of-importance/.
15. Pinola, Melanie. "The Science of Memory: Top 10 Proven Techniques to Remember More and Learn Faster." Zapier, Zapier, 10 July 2020, zapier.com/blog/better-memory/.
16. Saubers, Nadine. "First Aid." Metals Reference Book, 1976, pp. 1–4., doi:10.1016/b978-0-408-70627-8.50006-5.
17. Spencer, John. "8 Strategies to Keep Informational Reading Fun." Edutopia, George Lucas Educational Foundation, 2 Apr. 2015, www.edutopia.org/blog/strategies-keep-informational-reading-fun-john-spencer.
18. St. John Ambulance Guide to First Aid and CPR. (n.d.). Retrieved October 11, 2020, from https://books.google.ae/books?id=yU0GAAAACAAJ.
19. The Importance of Visual Communication, Digicast Productions, 23 Mar. 2014, youtu.be/Poudrd4AYks.
20. The Purpose, Content & Structure of Manuals.Study.com, study.com/academy/lesson/the-purpose-content-structure-of-manuals.html.
21. Wahl, Jordan. "Five eBook Formats and How to Find the Best Style for You." G2, learn.g2.com/eBook-formats.
22. Why is proper formatting of a document important? (n.d.). Retrieved October 10, 2020, from https://connectsus.com/help/faq/why-proper-formatting-document-important.

23. Maddison, Tasha, et al. Distributed Learning: Pedagogy and Technology in Online Information Literacy Instruction. Chandos Publishing, Cambridge, MA, 2017;2016;.
24. Basic First Aid Training UK (Updated 2020), Get Licensed, 7 May 2020, youtu.be/ErxKDbH-iiI.
25. First Aid – What You Need To Know, Rehealthify, 1 July 2014, youtu.be/A-Mf38Q-E1U.
26. Color Psychology In Web Design, GraVoc, 22 June 2015, youtu.be/r9gYdD-REI0.
27. MedicineNet.com. MedicineNet, MedicineNet, 13 June 2018, www.medicinenet.com/first_aid_witchdoctors_and_religious_knights/views.htm.
28. Daniels, S. (2019, April 26). Why is Visual Learning So Important? Retrieved September 4, 2020, from https://www.insightresources.org/2019/04/26/why-visual-learning-and-teaching/
29. First Aid Basics – Lesson One. (2020, June 09). Retrieved October 3, 2020, from https://nhcps.com/lesson/cpr-first-aid-first-aid-basics/
30. First Aid, CPR, and AED. (n.d.). Retrieved September 30, 2020, from https://books.google.ae/books? id=DcSR9DoZ3FQC31.First Aid Guide. (n.d.). Retrieved October 7, 2020, from https://books.google.ae/books? id=oQS4YSOHAo0C.

www.ingramcontent.com/pod-product-compliance
Lightning Source LLC
Chambersburg PA
CBHW040519220526
45473CB00012B/2912